Ninja Foodi Pressure Cooker Cookbook

365 Days Recipes for Easy and Tasty Meals

Maria Marshal

Table Of Contents

BREAKFAST
RECIPES
Green Tomato Chutney
(Ready in about 15 minutes | Servings 12)

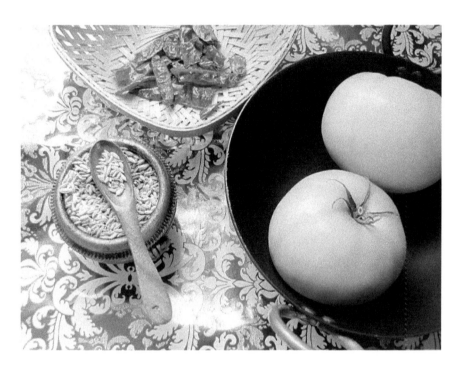

Ingredients

1. 2 pounds green tomatoes, diced

1. 2 garlic cloves, peeled and minced

1. 1 leek, thinly sliced

1. 1 jalapeño pepper, minced

1. 2 bell peppers, diced

1. 1/4 cup dried cherries

1. 1 tablespoon fresh ginger, grated

1. 3/4 cup brown sugar

1. 3/4 cup white wine

1. 3/4 teaspoon sea salt

Directions

1. Put all ingredients into the pressure cooking pot; stir to combine well. Cookon LOW pressure for 10 minutes. Remove from the heat and allow pressureto release gradually.

2. Place in a refrigerator before serving. You can spread your chutney overpizza crust if desired. Keep in your refrigerator for 2 months. Enjoy!

Homemade Peach Jam

(Ready in about 10 minutes | Servings 20)

Ingredients

1. 4 cups peaches, pitted, peeled and chopped

1. 4 cups sugar

1. 1 teaspoon orange juice

1. 1 teaspoon lemon juice

1. 1 (1 3⁄4-ounce) package dry pectin

Directions

1. Add the peaches, sugar, orange juice, and lemon juice to the pressurecooking pot. Stir until the ingredients are well combined.

2. Bring to low pressure and maintain pressure for 3 minutes. Remove fromthe heat and allow pressure to release.

3. Uncover and place over medium-high heat. Then, stir in the pectin; bringmixture to a boil, stirring often, for 1 minute.

4. Spoon into the sterilized glass containers. Keep in the freezer for up to 8 months.

Fruit Breakfast Risotto

(Ready in about 15 minutes | Servings 4)

Ingredients

1. 2 tablespoons margarine

1. 1 ½ cups rice

1. 1 large apple, cored and diced

1. 1 large pear, cored and diced

1. 1/2 teaspoon cinnamon

1. 1/8 teaspoon grated nutmeg

1. 1/8 teaspoon salt

1. 1/3 cup brown sugar

1. 1 cup apple juice

1. 3 cups milk

1. 1/2 cup dried cranberries

Directions

1. Melt the margarine in the pressure cooking pot for about 3 minutes. Addrice to the cooker; cook, stirring frequently, approximately 4 minutes.

2. Add the apple, pear, cinnamon, nutmeg, salt, and brown sugar. Add the apple juice and milk. Select HIGH pressure and cook 6 minutes. Then, turnoff your cooker and use a quick pressure release.

3. Afterwards, stir in dried cranberries. Serve topped with a splash of milk ifdesired.

FAST SNACKS RECIPES
Butternut Squash with Pine Nuts
(Ready in about 1 hour 15 minutes | Servings 6)

Ingredients

1. 1 butternut squash, peeled and sliced

1. 2 tablespoons extra-virgin olive oil

1. Salt and freshly ground pepper

1. 3 ½ ounces pine nuts

1. 1/2 cup green onions, chopped

1. 2 tablespoons tomato paste

1. 1 cup vegetable broth

1. 1 teaspoon grated lemon rind

1. 1/2 cup wine

1. 1/2 cup sharp cheese shavings

Directions

1. Begin by preheating your oven to 350 degrees F. Now spread the butternutsquash slices on a baking sheet; drizzle with 1 tablespoon of olive oil; sprinkle with salt and black pepper.

2. Cover with an aluminum foil; roast butternut squash slices until they are tender, or about 45 minutes. Add the squash to a food processor; puree untilit's smooth.

3. In the meantime, toast the pine nuts on a baking sheet for about 4 minutes.

4. Then, warm the remaining 1 tablespoon of olive oil in a pressure cooker.Add green onions and sauté until they are softened, 4 minutes. Add theroasted pine nuts and tomato paste; cook, stirring constantly, for about 2minutes.

5. Add the vegetable broth, lemon rind, and wine; cover and cook for 7minutes. Remove the lid and release the pressure.

6. Add the cooker back to medium heat; bring the contents to a boil. Cook forabout 4 minutes. Add the reserved squash puree; cook until it is warmed through. Serve with cheese shavings.

Zesty Appetizer Meatballs

(Ready in about 15 minutes | Servings 12)

Ingredients

1. 1/2 cup sugar

1. 2 tablespoons apple juice

1. 2/3 cup water

1. 1/3 cup white wine

1. 2 tablespoons tamari sauce

1. 2 tablespoons Worcestershire sauce

1. 2 tablespoons cornstarch

1. 1 pound ground beef

1. 2 cloves garlic, minced

1. 1 yellow onion, diced

1. 1/2 cup bread crumbs

Directions

1. Add the sugar, apple juice, water, white wine, tamari sauce, Worcestershiresauce, and cornstarch to a pressure cooker. Then, bring to a boil over HIGHheat.

2. Stir the mixture continuously until it has thickened; remove from heat.

3. In a mixing bowl, combine ground beef, garlic, yellow onion, and breadcrumbs; mix until it is well combined.

4. Roll the mixture into 12 equal meatballs; add meatballs to the sauce in thecooker. Lock the lid into place. Bring to high pressure; maintain pressure for 5 minutes.

5. Quick-release the pressure. Transfer to a large serving platter and servewarm.

Meatballs in Herbed Sauce

(Ready in about 15 minutes | Servings 12)

Ingredients

1. 2 tablespoons pineapple juice

1. 1 tablespoon maple syrup

1. 1 tablespoon dried thyme

1. 1 cup water

1. 2 tablespoons soy sauce

1. 1/2 pound ground pork

1. 1 pound extra lean ground beef

1. 2 cloves garlic, minced

1. 1 cup shallots, diced

1. 1/2 cup bread crumbs

1. Fresh parsley, for garnish

Directions

1. In your cooker, place pineapple juice, maple syrup, thyme, water, soysauce; stir to combine. Bring to a boil over HIGH heat.

2. Cook until the sauce has thickened; turn off the heat.

3. In a bowl, combine ground pork, ground beef, garlic, shallots, and breadcrumbs; mix until everything is incorporated.

4. Now shape the mixture into 12 equal meatballs; carefully transfer meatballsto the pressure cooker. Lock the lid into place and bring to HIGH pressure; maintain pressure for about 5 minutes.

5. Release pressure quickly. Transfer to a large serving platter. Sprinkle withfresh chopped parsley and serve warm.

Fast and Easy Carrot Coins

(Ready in about 5 minutes | Servings 6)

Ingredients

1. 1 cup water

1. 1 pound carrots, peeled and sliced into thick coins

Directions

1. Fill the cooker's base with water. Place the carrot coins in the steamerbasket; put the basket into the pressure cooker. Close the lid.

2. Turn the heat up to HIGH and maintain the pressure for 1 to 2 minutes atHIGH.

3. Afterwards, open the pressure cooker by releasing pressure. Replace to aserving platter and serve.

Butter and Maple Carrot Coins

(Ready in about 10 minutes | Servings 4)

Ingredients

1. 1 cup water

1. 1 pound carrots, trimmed and cut into thick coins

1. 2 tablespoons butter, softened

1. 1 tablespoon maple syrup

1. 1 teaspoon balsamic vinegar

1. Sea salt and freshly ground black pepper

1. 2 tablespoons fresh cilantro, chopped

Directions

1. Pour the water into your pressure
    cooker. Throw the carrots into the
    steamer basket and lay it in your
    pressure cooker.

2. Cover and maintain the pressure for 1 to 2
    minutes at HIGH. Then, open thepressure
    cooker by releasing pressure.

3. Warn butter in a saucepan over medium heat.
    Then, add carrots, and cookstirring
    occasionally, for about 3 minutes. Add maple
    syrup, balsamic vinegar, salt, and black
    pepper; cook for 1 more minute.

4. Remove to a serving platter and serve sprinkled
    with fresh cilantro. Enjoy!

LUNCH RECIPES
Creamed Asparagus Soup
(Ready in about 20 minutes | Servings 6)

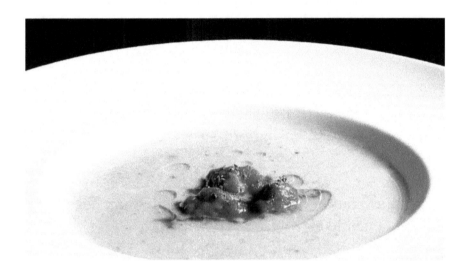

Ingredients

1. 2 tablespoons butter

1. 1 onion, diced

1. 2 pounds asparagus, trimmed and cut into pieces

1. 1 teaspoon garlic powder

1. 1 teaspoon salt

1. 1/2 teaspoon black pepper

1. 1⁄4 teaspoon cayenne pepper

1. 6 cups vegetable stock

1. 1⁄4 cup milk

1. 1 teaspoon lemon juice

Directions

1. Melt the butter in your pressure cooker; sauté the onion until tender andtranslucent. Add the asparagus, garlic powder, salt, black pepper, and cayenne pepper; sauté for 5 to 6 minutes.

2. Pour in the vegetable stock. Then, bring to HIGH pressure and cook forabout 5 minutes.

3. Remove from the heat and allow pressure to release naturally. Add the milkand lemon juice, and purée your soup in a food processor. Serve warm.

Lima Bean Soup

(Ready in about 20 minutes | Servings 6)

Ingredients

1. 2 cups dried lima beans

1. 2 tablespoons olive oil

1. 1/2 cup shallots, diced

1. 2 cloves garlic, minced

1. 1/2 cup water

1. 2 cups vegetable broth

1. Sea salt and ground black pepper, to taste

Directions

1. Pour water into medium-sized dish. Then, add lima beans and soak themovernight.

2. Warm olive oil in your pressure cooker; sauté the shallots until they aretender and golden brown. Then, add the garlic and cook for 1 minute longer.

3. Add the water, vegetable broth, and soaked lima beans to the cooker. Sealthe lid and continue to cook for 6 minutes. Remove from the heat and allowpressure to release gradually.

4. Purée the soup in a food processor; sprinkle with sea salt and ground blackpepper. Serve warm.

Potato Cheese Soup

(Ready in about 15 minutes | Servings 6)

Ingredients

1. 2 tablespoons butter

1. 1/2 cup red onion, chopped

1. 4 cups chicken broth

1. 3/4 teaspoon sea salt

1. 1/2 teaspoon black pepper

1. 1/4 teaspoon red pepper flakes, crushed

1. 6 cups potatoes, peeled and cubed

1. 2 tablespoons water

1. 2 tablespoons cornstarch

1. 1/2 cup Ricotta cheese, cut into cubes

1. 1 cup Cheddar cheese, shredded

1. 2 cups half and half

1. 1 cup frozen corn

Directions

1. Warm the butter in the pressure cooking pot. Sauté red onion for about 5minutes. Add 2 cups chicken broth, salt, pepper, and red pepper flakes.

2. Put the steamer basket into the pressure cooker. Add the potatoes to the basket. Lock the lid in place, cook 4 minutes at HIGH pressure. Carefullyremove the steamer basket from the pot.

3. In a small-sized bowl, dissolve cornstarch in water. Now add cornstarchmixture to the cooker, stirring often.

4. Add Ricotta cheese and Cheddar cheese. Stir until cheese is melted. Addremaining chicken broth, half and half, and corn. Cook for a few minuteslonger until the soup is heated through. Serve.

Garlicky Bean Soup

(Ready in about 15 minutes | Servings 8)

Ingredients

1. 2 cups dried white beans

1. 3 tablespoons olive oil

1. 1 medium-sized leek, sliced

1. 4 cloves garlic, minced

1. 2 cups water

1. 4 cups vegetable stock

1. 2 bay leaves

1. 1 teaspoon apple cider vinegar

1. Sea salt and freshly cracked black pepper, to taste

Directions

1. Soak your white beans for 8 hours or overnight in enough water to cover hem; drain and rinse.

2. In your pressure cooker, bring olive oil to temperature over medium heat.Now sauté the leek until it is golden brown. Add the garlic; continue sautéing for 1 minute more.

3. Pour in the water and vegetable stock; add bay leaves. Seal the lid and bringto HIGH pressure. Cook for about 10 minutes.

4. Remove the bay leaves; lastly, purée the soup and stir in the vinegar, salt,and black pepper. Ladle into individual dishes and serve warm.

DINNER RECIPES
Poached Salmon Fillets
(Ready in about 10 minutes | Servings 4)

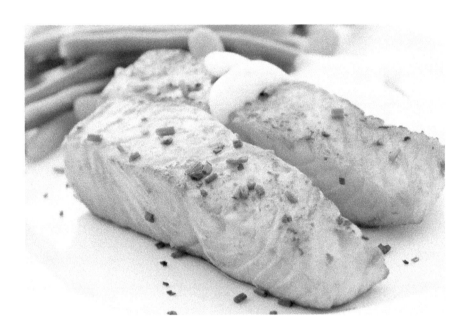

Ingredients

1. 3 tablespoons butter

1. 2 pounds salmon fillets

1. 1 cup chicken broth

1. 1 cup scallions, chopped

1. 2 cloves garlic, minced

1. Juice of 1 lime

1. 1 tablespoon fresh tarragon, chopped

1. Kosher salt and ground black pepper, to taste

Directions

1. Simply throw all the above ingredients in your pressure cooker.

2. Securely lock the pressure cooker's lid; set to 6 minutes on HIGH.

3. Then, release the cooker's pressure. Serve right now.

Spiced Lemony Scallops

(Ready in about 10 minutes | Servings 4)

Ingredients

1. 2 tablespoons olive oil

1. 1 onion, thinly sliced

1. 1 red bell pepper, seeded and sliced

1. 1 jalapeño pepper, seeded and chopped

1. 2 tomatoes, diced

1. 1 tablespoon chopped fresh oregano

1. 1 teaspoon granulated garlic

1. 1/3 cup chicken stock

1. 1 ½ pounds sea scallops

1. 1 small-sized lemon, freshly squeezed

1. Salt and ground black pepper, to taste

Directions

1. Warm olive oil over medium-high heat. Then, sauté the onion, bell pepper,and jalapeño pepper until they are tender.

2. Add tomatoes, oregano, granulated garlic, and chicken stock to the cooker;stir to combine.

3. Top with the scallops. Drizzle with lemon juice; salt and pepper to taste.

4. Cover the cooker and set for 2 minutes on HIGH. Serve immediately.

Flaky Tilapia Fillets

(Ready in about 10 minutes | Servings 2)

Ingredients

1. 2 tilapia fillets

1. Salt and black pepper, to taste

1. 1 teaspoon garlic powder

1. 2 sprigs thyme

1. 1 sprig rosemary

1. 2 slices lemon

1. 2 tablespoons butter, softened

Directions

1. Prepare 2 squares of parchment paper.

2. Lay a fillet in the center of each square of parchment paper. Sprinkle withsalt, black pepper, and garlic powder.

3. Sprinkle with thyme and rosemary. Drizzle with lemon and butter. Close upparchment paper around the tilapia fillets in order to form two packets.

4. Next, place a trivet at the bottom of the cooker. Pour 1 cup of water into thecooker. Lay the packets on the trivet.

5. Cover the cooker with the lid and set for 5 minutes on HIGH. Serve rightaway!

DESSERT RECIPES
Quinoa Pudding with Walnuts
(Ready in about 10 minutes | Servings 6)

Ingredients

1. 2 ¼ cups water

1. 1 ½ cups quinoa

1. 1/4 cup agave nectar

1. 1/2 teaspoon vanilla

1. 1/4 teaspoon nutmeg, preferably freshly grated

1. 1/2 teaspoon cinnamon powder

1. Chopped walnuts, toasted

Directions

1. Add the water, quinoa, agave nectar, vanilla, nutmeg, and cinnamonpowder to the pressure cooking pot.

2. Select HIGH pressure and cook for 5 minutes. Next, turn your cooker off;use a Quick Pressure Release to release pressure.

3. Fluff the quinoa and serve warm with the toasted walnuts.

Old-Fashioned Cocoa Custard

(Ready in about 10 minutes | Servings 4)

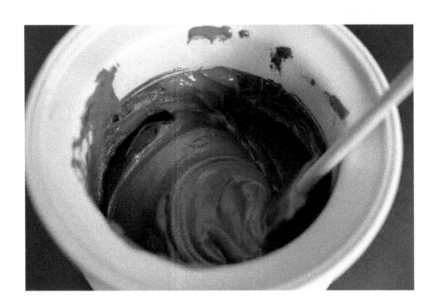

Ingredients

1. 2 cups milk

1. 2 whole eggs

1. 1/3 cup sugar

1. 1 tablespoon cocoa powder

1. 1/2 teaspoon vanilla essence

1. 1 cup water

Directions

1. Start by scalding the milk; then, allow the milk to slightly cool.

2. Add the eggs, sugar, cocoa powder, milk, and vanilla to a mixing bowl; stirto combine well. Pour the mixture into 4 custard cups; cover cups with analuminum foil.

3. Add water to your cooker's base; now put trivet and steamer basket into thecooker. Place prepared custard cups in the steamer basket.

4. Lock the lid in place; cook for 3 minutes on HIGH pressure. Let thepressure drop using the quick-release method. Serve chilled.

Summer Caramel Custard

(Ready in about 10 minutes | Servings 4)

Ingredients

1. 2 cups milk

1. 3 eggs yolks

1. 1/3 cup caster sugar

1. 1/2 teaspoon vanilla paste

1. 1/4 teaspoon freshly grated nutmeg

1. A dash of cinnamon powder

1. 1 cup water

Directions

1. Begin by scalding the milk and allow it to slightly cool.

2. In a mixing bowl, combine together the egg yolks, caster sugar, vanilla paste, nutmeg, and cinnamon; add reserved milk; whisk well to combine.Pour the mixture into 4 custard cups; cover cups with a foil.

3. Pour the water into the cooker. Then, lay a rack and steamer basket in thecooker. Lay prepared custard cups in the steamer basket.

4. Cover with the lid and cook for 3 minutes on HIGH. Let the pressure dropusing the quick-release method. Transfer to a refrigerator to chill before serving.

Stewed Prunes and Dried Apricots

(Ready in about 10 minutes | Servings 6)

Ingredients

1. 1 cup water

1. 1 cup red wine

1. 3/4 cup brown sugar

1. 1 vanilla bean

1. 3-4 cloves

1. 1 cinnamon stick

1. 2 lemon slices

1. 1/2 pound prunes

1. 1/2 pound dried apricots

Directions

1. In your cooker, mix together the water, red wine, brown sugar, vanilla bean,cloves, cinnamon stick, and lemon slices. Bring to a boil; let it simmer untilbrown sugar dissolves.

2. Add the prunes and apricots. Cook for 4 minutes on HIGH pressure. Servewarm or at room temperature. Enjoy!

Winter Stewed Fruits

(Ready in about 10 minutes | Servings 6)

Ingredients

1. 1/2 cup red wine

1. 1 ½ cups water

1. 1/2 cup agave syrup

1. 3-4 cloves

1. 2 cinnamon sticks

1. 1/2 teaspoon vanilla essence

1. 1/2 orange, sliced

1. 1/2 pound dried apples

1. 1/4 pound dried prunes

1. 1/4 pound dried figs

Directions

1. In your cooker, mix together the wine, water, agave syrup, cloves,cinnamon sticks, vanilla, and orange. Bring the mixture to a boil.

2. Add dried fruits. Cook for 4 minutes on HIGH. Serve with vanilla ice creamif desired.

INSTANT POT

BREAKFAST RECIPES
Bacon and Vegetable Breakfast
(Ready in about 10 minutes | Servings 4)

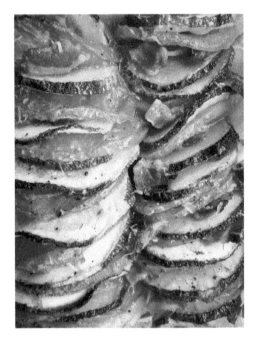

Ingredients

1. 2 tablespoons canola oil

1. 3 slices bacon, chopped

1. 1 cup cabbage, shredded

1. 1 red bell pepper, thinly sliced

1. Salt and black pepper, to taste

Directions

1. Press "Sauté" and add the canola oil to melt. Add the rest of the ingredients.

2. Seal the lid and choose "Manual" for 5 minutes. Serve over bread or cookedquinoa.

Breakfast Bean Casserole

(Ready in about 30 minutes | Servings 8)

Ingredients

1. 1 pound lima beans

1. 1/2 teaspoon sea salt

1. 1 bay leaf

1. 3/4 cup butter

1. 1/4 cup sugar

1. 1 teaspoon granulated garlic

1. 1 teaspoon mustard

1. 1 teaspoon sea salt

1. 1 cup sour cream

1. Fresh chopped chives, for garnish

Directions

1. First, soak lima beans with 10 cups of water. Then, add salt and bay leaf,and press "Manual". Cook for 4 minutes under HIGH pressure.

2. Press "Keep Warm" button and leave it for 10 minutes; next, quick releasepressure.

3. Drain lima beans; add them back to the pot. Next, add the remainingingredients, except for chives.

4. Cook for 10 minutes on "Manual" under HIGH pressure. Serve garnishedwith fresh chives. Enjoy!

Bean and Apple Salad

(Ready in about 45 minutes | Servings 8)

Ingredients

1. 10 ounces red kidney beans

1. 3 cloves garlic, finely minced

1. 1 onion, chopped fine

1. 1 crisp apple, cored and diced

1. 1/4 cup brown sugar

1. 1 teaspoon sea salt

1. 1 tablespoon fresh basil

1. 1 tablespoon dry oregano

1. 1 teaspoon red pepper flakes, crushed

1. Black pepper, to taste

Directions

1. Soak kidney beans overnight.

2. Then, transfer soaked beans to the inner pot along with the remainingingredients. Add water (2 inches above the top of beans).

3. Cook for 45 minutes. Serve chilled.

Rice Pudding with Prunes and Dates

(Ready in about 20 minutes | Servings 6)

Ingredients

1. 1 ½ cups Arborio rice

1. 1/2 cup sugar

1. 1 tablespoon maple syrup

1. A pinch of kosher salt

1. 5 cups whole milk

1. 2 eggs

1. 1 cup evaporated milk

1. 1/2 cup prunes, chopped

1. 1/2 cup dates, pitted and chopped

1. Cinnamon powder to taste

1. Anise seeds, to taste

Directions

1. In the inner pot, combine Arborio rice, sugar, maple syrup, kosher salt, and5 cups of whole milk.

2. Now choose the "Sauté" button; bring to a boil, stirring continuously todissolve the sugar. Then, lock the lid in place. Press the "Rice" button.

3. Meanwhile, whisk the eggs and evaporated milk. Afterwards, perform thequick-pressure release. Stir in the egg-milk mixture, prunes, dates, cinnamon, and anise.

4. Press the "Sauté". Cook uncovered until the pudding starts to boil. Serve atroom temperature.

LUNCH RECIPES
Potato Leek Soup with Cremini Mushrooms
(Ready in about 20 minutes | Servings 10)

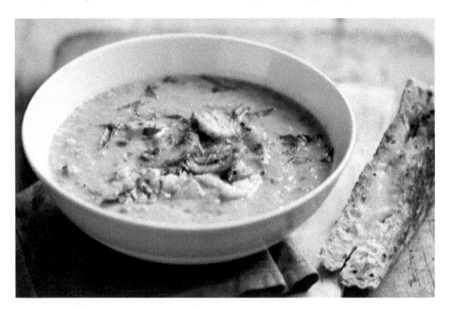

Ingredients

1. 2 small-sized leeks, trimmed and sliced

1. 2 cloves garlic, minced

1. 8 cups water, boiling

1. 2 pounds potatoes, peeled and cubed

1. 2 parsnips, peeled and diced

1. 3 medium-sized carrots, peeled and diced

1. 1 cup cremini mushrooms, roughly chopped

1. 1 teaspoon marjoram

1. 1/2 teaspoon fennel seeds

1. Salt and black pepper, to your liking

1. 2 cups unsweetened coconut milk

Directions

1. Choose "Sauté" function; now sauté the leeks and garlic approximately 5minutes, adding boiling water as needed.

2. Add the rest of the ingredients, except for coconut milk. Lock the cooker's lid in place; cook under HIGH pressure for about 6 minutes.

3. After that, allow the cooker's pressure to come down gradually andnaturally. Pour in the coconut milk.

4. Mix your soup with an immersion blender. Adjust the seasonings, and servewarm topped with nutritional yeast if desired.

Creamy and Cheesy Cauliflower Soup

(Ready in about 15 minutes | Servings 8)

Ingredients

1. 8 cups cauliflower florets

1. 1 cup boiling water

1. 3 cups vegetable broth

1. 2 garlic cloves, minced

1. 1/2 cup shallots, chopped

1. Sea salt and ground black pepper, to your liking

1. 1 teaspoon paprika

1. 1 teaspoon marjoram

1. 1 teaspoon cumin powder

1. 1 cup Cheddar cheese, shredded

Directions

1. Simply throw all the ingredients, except for Cheddar cheese, into yourcooker.

2. Next, place the lid on, and choose "MANUAL"; set time to 6 minutes.Open the cooker.

3. Process the soup in a blender or a food processor, working in batches. Ladleinto individual bowls and serve topped with shredded Cheddar cheese. Enjoy!

Zucchini and Summer Squash Soup

(Ready in about 25 minutes | Servings 8)

Ingredients

1. 1 onion, peeled and chopped

1. 4 zucchinis, shredded

1. 4 yellow summer squashes, shredded

1. 2 serrano peppers, diced

1. 1 orange bell pepper, diced

1. 1 (12-ounce) package silken tofu, pressed

1. 1 cup boiling water

1. 1 cup vegetable stock

1. 1 tablespoon chili powder

1. 1 teaspoon cumin powder

1. 1 teaspoon smoked paprika

Directions

1. Add the onion to your cooker. Press "Sauté" button; then, sauté the onionsuntil tender and translucent.

2. Add the rest of the ingredients and press "Soup" button.

3. Remove the lid according to manufacturer's directions. Allow to cool slightly; mix with an immersion blender.

4. Serve in individual bowls topped with fresh chopped cilantro. Enjoy!

Beef and Kale Stew with Noodles

(Ready in about 25 minutes | Servings 8)

Ingredients

1. 2 tablespoons butter

1. 1/2 pound ground beef

1. 1 teaspoon dried basil leaves

1. 1/2 teaspoon dried thyme

1. 1/2 teaspoon marjoram

1. 1/2 teaspoon cayenne pepper

1. Salt and black pepper, to taste

1. 1 onion, diced

1. 3 carrots, diced

1. 1/2 cup white wine

1. 2 Roma tomatoes, seeded and chopped

1. 8 cups bone broth

1. 2 large handfuls kale, chopped

1. 8 ounces noodles

Directions

1. Set your cooker to "Sauté". Now melt butter; then, add the ground beef andall of the seasonings. Cook till the meat has browned.

2. Add the onion and carrot, and cook for about 7 minutes. Pour in the wine todeglaze the pan.

3. Add the rest of the ingredients, and stir to combine. Serve topped with freshcilantro if desired.

DINNER RECIPES
Pasta with Beef and Mushrooms
(Ready in about 20 minutes | Servings 4)

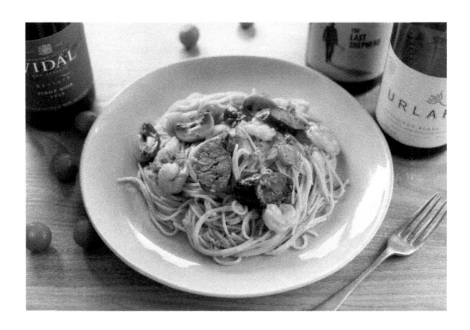

Ingredients

1. 1 tablespoon olive oil

1. 1 pound lean ground beef

1. 1 onion

1. 2 garlic cloves, minced

1. 2 pounds tomato puree

1. 1 ½ cups mushrooms, chopped

1. 1 teaspoon dried basil leaves

1. 1/2 teaspoon dried oregano

1. Salt and black pepper, ground

1. 1 cup dried egg noodles

Directions

1. Cook ground beef in olive oil using the "Sauté" function on your cooker. Then, add the onions and garlic; sauté until they're tender.

2. Add the rest of the ingredients. Pressure cook for 7 minutes. Serve andenjoy!

71

Easiest Chicken Risotto

(Ready in about 20 minutes | Servings 4)

Ingredients

1. 1 stick butter, at room temperature

1. 1 red onion, chopped

1. 3 garlic cloves, chopped

1. 1 pound chicken, diced

1. 2 cups rice

1. 1 cup white wine

1. 4 cups chicken stock

1. 1 teaspoon rosemary

1. Salt and freshly ground black pepper, to your liking

1. Chopped fresh parsley, for garnish

Directions

1. Use "Sauté" function to preheat your cooker. Now warm the butter, andcook the onion, garlic, and chicken for about 2 minutes.

2. Stir in rice and wine. Add chicken stock, rosemary, salt, and black pepper.Use "Manual" mode, and adjust the time to 12 minutes. Give it another good stir. Now seal the lid.

3. Serve topped with fresh parsley. Enjoy!

Pancetta Risotto with Feta Cheese

(Ready in about 20 minutes | Servings 4)

Ingredients

1. 1 tablespoon olive oil

1. 1 leek, chopped

1. 2 garlic cloves, chopped

1. 1 ½ cups pancetta, diced

1. 2 cups rice

1. 5 cups chicken stock

1. 1 tablespoon apple cider vinegar

1. 1 teaspoon dried thyme

1. 1/2 teaspoon dried basil

1. 1/2 teaspoon dried dill weed

1. 1 teaspoon mustard powder

1. Salt and freshly ground black pepper, to your liking

1. Feta cheese, crumbled

Directions

1. Press "Sauté" button and heat the oil; sauté the leek and garlic until they aretender.

2. Stir in the pancetta, rice, and chicken stock. Add apple cider vinegar,thyme, basil, dill weed, and mustard powder.

3. Next, press "Manual" button; set the time to 12 minutes. Season with saltand black pepper; stir to combine well and cover with the lid.

4. Serve topped with crumbled Feta cheese. Serve right away.

Herby Pasta with Meat and Mushrooms

(Ready in about 30 minutes | Servings 4)

Ingredients

1. 2 tablespoons canola oil

1. 2 cloves garlic, minced

1. 1 large-sized onion, chopped fine

1. 1 pound ground pork

1. 1 pound ground beef

1. 1 teaspoon sea salt

1. 1/2 teaspoon ground black pepper

1. 1/2 teaspoon red pepper flakes

1. 1/2 teaspoon dried dill weed

1. 1/2 teaspoon dried basil

1. 1 teaspoon dried sage

1. 2 small cans mushrooms, sliced

1. 1 jar pasta sauce

1. 1 pound uncooked pasta

1. 3 cups chicken broth

1. 1 cup dry wine

Directions

1. Press "Sauté" button and warm canola oil. Sauté the garlic, onion, pork, andbeef until browned.

2. Add the remaining ingredients. Stir until everything is well combined. Sealthe cooker's lid and cook for 20 minutes. Release the pressure manually.

3. Serve with Mozzarella cheese if desired. Serve.

FAST SNACKS
Mom's Famous Kale Humus
(Ready in about 35 minutes | Servings 12)

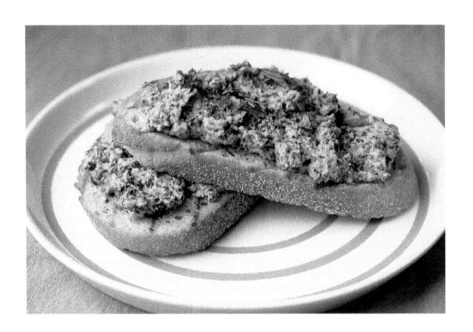

Ingredients

1. 4 cups water

1. 1 cup garbanzo beans

1. 1 cup packed kale leaves

1. 2 garlic cloves, minced

1. 1 tablespoon salt

1. 2 tablespoons tahini

1. 1/4 cup extra-virgin olive oil

Directions

1. Add water and garbanzo beans to your Instant Pot.

2. Secure the lid; choose "Manual" function and cook for 25 minutes. Turn offthe heat. Now drain your garbanzo beans and transfer them to a food processor.

3. Add kale, garlic, salt, and tahini. Puree until creamy and uniform. Then, gradually pour olive oil in a thin stream. Continue mixing till it reaches your desired texture.

4. Serve with dippers of choice, such as bread sticks, crackers, veggie sticks,and so on.

Vegan Spinach
Dip

(Ready in about 10 minutes | Servings 12)

Ingredients

1. 1 package (10-ounce) frozen chopped spinach, thawed

1. 1 cup silken lite tofu

1. 1 cup Vegan mayonnaise

1. 1 teaspoon Dijon mustard

1. 1/2 teaspoon salt

1. 1/4 teaspoon ground black pepper

1. Lemon zest, for garnish

Directions

1. Set trivet in your Instant Pot. Place all the ingredients, except for lemon zest, in a baking dish; now stir with a spoon to combine well. Next, wrapthe baking dish in a foil.

2. Make a foil sling and place it on prepared trivet. Lay the baking dish on thefoil sling. Secure the cooker's lid; press "Manual" and set the timer to 8 minutes. Serve sprinkled with lemon zest.

Perfect Pumpkin Hummus

(Ready in about 35 minutes | Servings 16)

Ingredients

1. 4 cups water

1. 1 cup chickpeas

1. 1 cup canned pumpkin puree

1. 2 garlic cloves, minced

1. A pinch crushed sea salt

1. 1 tablespoon fresh lemon juice

1. 2 tablespoons tahini

1. 1/4 cup olive oil

1. Paprika, for garnish

Directions

1. Add water and chickpeas to the Instant Pot.

2. Cover your cooker and select "Manual" mode;
   cook for 25 minutes. Turnoff the cooker.
   Now drain your chickpeas; transfer them to a
   food processor.

3. Add pumpkin puree, garlic, salt, lemon, and
   tahini. Puree until the mixturebecomes
   uniform. Slowly add the oil in a thin stream.
   Continue mixing until you create a silken
   texture.

4. Sprinkle with paprika; you can decorate
   hummus with a few wholechickpeas if
   desired; serve with veggie sticks.

Chili Pumpkin Hummus

(Ready in about 35 minutes | Servings 16)

Ingredients

1. 1 cup chickpeas

1. 4 cups water

1. 1 shallot, peeled and finely minced

1. 2 garlic cloves, minced

1. 1 cup canned pumpkin puree

1. 1 teaspoon Dukkah spice blend

1. 3/4 teaspoon crushed sea salt

1. 1/2 tsp chipotle chili powder

1. Pinch of ground cardamom

1. 1 tablespoon soy sauce

1. 1 tablespoon lemon juice

1. 1 teaspoon lemon zest

1. 1 tablespoon cilantro paste

1. 2 tablespoons tahini

1. 1/4 cup olive oil

1. Toasted pumpkin seeds, for garnish

Directions

1. Select "Manual" function, and cook chickpeas in water for 25 minutes.Carefully open the cooker and drain the cooked chickpeas; transfer chickpeas to your food processor.

2. Stir in the shallot, garlic, pumpkin puree, Dukkah spice blend, and sea salt.Mix to combine.

3. Now add chili powder, cardamom, soy sauce, lemon juice, lemon zest, cilantro paste and tahini. Puree until everything is well combined. Slowlyand gradually add olive oil. Continue mixing until everything is well incorporated.

4. Serve sprinkled with pumpkin seeds and enjoy!

Cremini Mushrooms and Asparagus Appetizer

(Ready in about 10 minutes | Servings 6)

Ingredients

1. 1 cup sliced cremini mushrooms

1. 1 cup scallions, thinly sliced

1. 1 cup asparagus, chopped

1. 1 teaspoon cumin powder

1. 1 teaspoon garlic powder

1. 2 tablespoons water

1. Sea salt and ground black pepper, to your liking

Directions

1. Click "Sauté" and cook the mushrooms and scallions until tender or forabout 1 minute.

2. Add the rest of the ingredients. Lock the lid and cook on HIGH pressure;set the timer to 2 minutes. Quick release pressure.

3. Transfer to a large serving platter and serve.

DESSERT RECIPES
Cheesecake with Raspberry Sauce
(Ready in about 35 minutes | Servings 10)

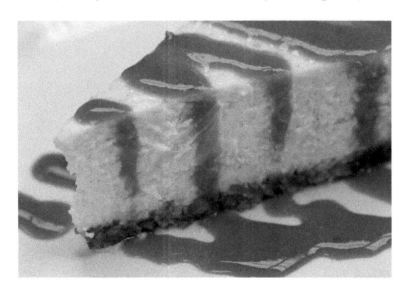

Ingredients

1. 1 ¼ cups graham cracker crumbs

1. 5 tablespoons butter, at room temperature

1. 1 pound cream cheese

1. 1/2 cup sugar

1. 2 eggs

1. 1/4 cup sour cream

1. 1 tablespoon lemon zest, finely grated

1. 2 tablespoons flour

1. 1/2 teaspoon vanilla extract

1. Raspberry sauce, for garnish

Directions

1. First, add 2 cups of water to your cooker. Now set a rack into the cooker.

2. Mix graham cracker crumbs and the butter until everything is well combined. Grease the inside of your springform pan and press the crumbmixture into the bottom of the pan.

3. In a food processor, beat the cream cheese together with sugar; process until smooth. With the processor running, slowly add the eggs (one at a time). Now stir in sour cream, lemon zest, flour, and vanilla. Process until everything is well mixed.

4. Pour the batter into the pan. Next, using a foil, form a sling that will holdthe pan. Lower the springform pan into the cooker. Lock the lid.

5. Select "Manual" key. Cook at HIGH pressure for 25 minutes. Uncover andremove the pan. Allow to cool completely before serving. Serve with raspberry sauce.

Frozen Lime Cheesecake

(Ready in about 35 minutes + chilling time | Servings 10)

Ingredients

1. 1 ¼ cups digestive biscuits, crumbled

1. 5 tablespoons butter, at room temperature

1. 1 pound full-fat cream cheese

1. 1/3 cup caster sugar

1. 2 whole eggs, room temperature

1. 1/4 cup sour cream

1. Zest and juice from 2 limes

1. 1 tablespoon lemon zest, finely grated

1. 2 tablespoons flour

1. 1/2 teaspoon grated ginger

1. 1/2 teaspoon anise seeds

1. 1/2 teaspoon vanilla extract

Directions

1. In a bowl, combine crumbled biscuits and butter. Lightly grease the insideof a springform pan with non-stick cooking spray. Now press the biscuitmixture into the bottom of the spring-form pan.

2. Next, add 2 cups of water to your Instant Pot. Now lay trivet at the bottomof the cooker.

3. In a food processor, mix the cream cheese together with caster sugar;process until creamy and smooth. Fold in the eggs, one at a time.

4. Add the rest of the ingredients. Pulse until everything is well blended.

5. Pour the batter into the springform pan. Cook at HIGH pressure; set the timer to 25 minutes. Wrap your cheesecake in a foil and freeze overnight.Serve.

Spicy Berry Compote

(Ready in about 10 minutes | Servings 8)

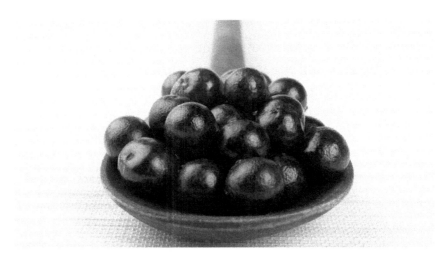

Ingredients

1. 1 cup red currants

1. 1 cup black currants

1. 1 cup strawberries

1. 4 cups water

1. 1/2 cup sugar

1. 1/2 teaspoon cardamom pods

1. 1/2 teaspoon cloves

1. 1 teaspoon cinnamon powder

1. 1 vanilla pod

Directions

1. Simply throw the ingredients in an ovenproof dish.

2. Set trivet into your cooker. Place the dish on the trivet. Choose "STEAM"button and cook for 5 minutes. Then, use the steam release.

3. Serve warm or at room temperature with vanilla ice cream if desired.